I0223365

56 Common Cold Dessert Solutions:

Dessert Recipes That Will Help You Prevent And Cure the Common Cold without the Use of Pills or Medicine

By

Joe Correa CSN

COPYRIGHT

© 2016 Live Stronger Faster Inc.

All rights reserved

Reproduction or translation of any part of this work beyond that permitted by section 107 or 108 of the 1976 United States Copyright Act without the permission of the copyright owner is unlawful.

This publication is designed to provide accurate and authoritative information in regard to the subject matter covered. It is sold with the understanding that neither the author nor the publisher is engaged in rendering medical advice. If medical advice or assistance is needed, consult with a doctor. This book is considered a guide and should not be used in any way detrimental to your health. Consult with a physician before starting this nutritional plan to make sure it's right for you.

ACKNOWLEDGEMENTS

This book is dedicated to my friends and family that have had mild or serious illnesses so that you may find a solution and make the necessary changes in your life.

56 Common Cold Dessert Solutions:

Dessert Recipes That Will Help You Prevent And Cure the Common Cold without the Use of Pills or Medicine

By

Joe Correa CSN

CONTENTS

ABOUT THE AUTHOR

After years of Research, I honestly believe in the positive effects that proper nutrition can have over the body and mind. My knowledge and experience has helped me live healthier throughout the years and which I have shared with family and friends. The more you know about eating and drinking healthier, the sooner you will want to change your life and eating habits.

Nutrition is a key part in the process of being healthy and living longer so get started today. The first step is the most important and the most significant.

INTRODUCTION

56 Common Cold Dessert Solutions: Dessert Recipes That Will Help You Prevent And Cure the Common Cold without the Use of Pills or Medicine

By Joe Correa CSN

The common cold is a viral disease of the upper respiratory tract, primarily the nose, throat, and sinuses. There are over 200 known viruses that cause the common cold and they are mostly spread through the air or in direct contact with people who have already been affected by it. These rather tiring viruses usually attack during the cold winter months and affect all age groups. The average adult gets two to four colds per year, while children get six to eight because of their weaker immune system. Besides having a weaker immune system, some other lifestyle factors can greatly contribute to the body's inability to protect itself. Among the most important ones are pshychological stress and lack of sleep.

The common cold has been with us since ancient times. People are fighting it every single year for their entire life. The most common symptoms are a runny nose, sneezing, sore throat, mild headache, and generally feeling weak. These symptoms are nothing else but the body's response to the infection.

Scientific research shows the strong relation between a healthy diet full of different nutrients and the common cold. This is quite expected, proper nutrition boosts up our immune system making it more resistant to different viruses. The stronger your immune system means a stronger body and fewer colds. As simple as that! Boosting your immune system is a never ending process that starts the moment we are born through our mother's milk. It continues with a nutrient-rich diet every single day for the rest of our lives.

A proper, healthy diet must include plenty of fruits and vegetables, beans, legumes, nuts, and seeds because these foods are abundant in different vitamins and minerals that are crucial for building up the immune system and the proper functioning of the entire organism.

This cookbook was created with a single purpose, to give you plenty of different and tasty ideas on how to combine some of the healthiest foods and prepare a meal that will be powerful yet tasty. A collection of healthy recipes full of green vegetables, lean meat, fruits, nuts, and seeds is big enough to provide a unique meal for everyones taste buds!

Let this book be your guide on how to eat healthy and live a cold-free life!

56 COMMON COLD DESSERT SOLUTIONS: DESSERT RECIPES THAT WILL HELP YOU PREVENT AND CURE THE COMMON COLD WITHOUT THE USE OF PILLS OR MEDICINE

1. Warm Winter Compote

Ingredients:

1 lb of fresh figs, chopped

7 oz of Turkish figs, chopped

7 oz of fresh cherries

7 oz of plums, pitted and halved

4 oz of raisins

3 large apples, cored and chopped

3 tbsp of cornstarch

1 tsp of cinnamon, ground

1 tbsp of cloves

1 large lemon, juiced

3 cups of water

Preparation:

Combine all ingredients in a deep pot. Add more water to adjust the thickness of the compote. Cover with a lid and cook for 1 hour over a medium-low temperature. Remove from the heat and transfer to a serving bowls.

Serve warm.

Nutrition information per serving: Kcal: 385, Protein: 3.1g, Carbs: 100g, Fats: 1.1g

2. Brussel Sprout Soup

Ingredients:

1lb of Brussel sprouts, halved

7oz fresh baby spinach, torn

1 tsp of sea salt

1 cup of whole milk

3 tbsp of sour cream

1 tbsp of fresh celery, finely chopped

2 cups of water

1 tbsp of butter

Preparation:

Melt the butter in a large nonstick saucepan over a medium-high temperature. Add Brussel sprouts, baby spinach, and ½ cup of water. Cook for 5 minutes, stirring occasionaly.

Now, add milk, celery, and 2 cups of water. Stir well and cook for 10 minutes. Transfer the soup to the food processor and blend until smooth. Return the soup to the saucepan and stir in the sour cream. Cover with a lid and cook for 40 minutes on a medium-low temperature. Sprinkle with some salt and give it a good stir. Remove from the heat and serve warm.

Nutrition information per serving: Kcal: 194, Protein: 10.6g, Carbs: 21.7g, Fats: 9.8g

3. Green Citrus Smoothie

Ingredients:

2 cups of baby spinach, chopped

1 large banana, chopped

½ cup of orange juice, freshly squeezed

1 tbsp of honey, raw

1 medium-sized lemon, peeled and chopped

1 tsp of ginger, ground

2 tbsp of flaxseeds

Preparation:

Combine banana, lemon, orange juice, ginger, honey, and flaxseeds in a blender. Blend until smooth, then add spinach. Add water to adjust the thickness if needed. Re-blend for 1 minute and transfer to a serving glasses. Serve immediately.

Nutrition information per serving: Kcal: 167, Protein: 3.4g, Carbs: 34.4g, Fats: 2.7g

4. Garlic Meatballs

Ingredients:

1lb of lean beef, ground

7oz white rice

2 small onions, finely chopped

2 garlic cloves, crushed

1 large egg, beaten

1 large potato, peeled and sliced

3 tbsp of olive oil

1 tsp of salt

Preparation:

Combine meat, rice, finely chopped onions, crushed garlic, beaten egg, and salt in a large bowl. Stir well with spatula or with hands to combine. Shape the mixture into 15-20 meatballs, depending on the size.

Grease the bottom of a deep pot with 3 tablespoons of olive oil. Make the first layer with slice potatoes and top with meatballs.

Cover with a lid and cook for about 2 hours over a low temperature. Serve with yogurt or cream cheese. However, this is optional.

Nutrition information per serving: Kcal: 468, Protein: 33.4g, Carbs: 47.6g, Fats: 15.3g

5. Creamy Beetroot Salad

Ingredients:

2 medium-sized beetroots, trimmed and chopped

1 cup of kefir

3 cups of arugula, chopped

1 cup of spinach, chopped

½ cup of orange juice

2 tbsp of lemon juice

2 tbsp of olive oil

¼ cup of pistachios, roughly chopped

½ tsp of salt

¼ tsp of black pepper, ground

1 tsp of lime zest

Preparation:

Combine orange juice, lemon juice, oil, pistachios, salt, and pepper in a large bowl. Set aside to allow flavors to mingle.

Place the beetroots in a pot of boiling water. Sprinkle with salt and cook for 10 minutes, or until soften. Remove from the heat and drain well. Transfer into the marinade bowl and set aside for at least 1 hour.

Meanwhile, combine kefir, arugula, and spinach in a separate bowl toss well. Spoon about 2 tablespoons of the mixture on a serving plate and top with beetroot mixture. Repeat the remaining process and drizzle with remaining marinade. Sprinkle with lime zest and serve.

Nutrition information per serving: Kcal: 167, Protein: 6.0g, Carbs: 14.7g, Fats: 9.8g

6. Moroccan Chickpea Soup

Ingredients:

14 oz of chickpeas, soaked

2 large carrots, finely chopped

2 small onions, peeled and finely chopped

2 large tomatoes, peeled and finely chopped

3 tbsp of tomato paste

2 cups of vegetable broth

3 tbsp of extra-virgin olive oil

1 tsp of salt

A handful of fresh parsley, finely chopped

Preparation:

Soak the chickpeas overnight. Rinse, drain, and set aside.

Preheat the oil in a deep pot over a medium-high temperature. Place the rinsed chickpeas, chopped onions, carrot, and finely chopped tomatoes. Stir wel and cook for 2 minutes.

Pour the vegetable broth. Add water to adjust the thickness if needed. Stir in the tomato paste and sprinkle with some salt to taste. Cover with a lid and reduce the heat to low. Cook for about 1-2 hours and remove from the heat. Sprinkle with parsley before serving.

Nutrition information per serving: Kcal: 420, Protein: 18.9g, Carbs: 58.6g, Fats: 14.3g

7. Cold Cauliflower Salad

Ingredients:

1 lb of cauliflower florets, chopped

1 lb of broccoli, chopped

4 garlic cloves, crushed

2 tbsp of olive oil

1 tsp of salt

2 tbsp of lemon juice

½ tsp of Cayenne pepper, ground

1 tbsp of dry rosemary, crushed

Preparation:

Rinse and drain the vegetables.

Preheat the oil in a large skillet over a medium-high temperature. Add garlic and stir-fry until translucent. Add broccoli and cauliflower and cook for 5 minutes, stirring constantly. Remove from the heat and transfer to a salad bowl. Drizzle with lemon juice and stir well. Sprinkle with Cayenne pepper, rosemary, and salt. Chill well before serving.

Nutrition information per serving: Kcal: 182, Protein: 5.7g, Carbs: 15.1g, Fats: 13.2g

8. Classic Ragout Soup

Ingredients:

1 lb of lamb chop, boneless and cut into bite-sized pieces

1 cup of peas

4 medium-sized carrots, finely chopped

3 small onions, finely chopped

1 large potato, peeled and finely chopped

1 large tomato, diced

3 tbsp of olive oil

1 tbsp of Cayenne pepper, ground

1 tsp of salt

½ tsp of black pepper, ground

Preparation:

Place peas, carrots, and potatoes in a deep pot. Add enough water to cover the ingredients and bring it to a boil. Cook for 5 minutes and remove from the heat. Drain well and set aside.

Preheat the oil in a large skillet over a medium-high temperature. Add onions, and stir-fry until translucent. Add meat chops and cook for 20 minutes, or until nicely brown. Add pre-cooked vegetables, tomato, and ½ cup of water. Sprinkle with Cayenne pepper, salt, and pepper to taste. Reduce the lid to low and cook for 10 minutes.

Nutrition information per serving: Kcal: 307, Protein: 24.9g, Carbs: 23.3g, Fats: 13.2g

9. Orange Ginger Smoothie

Ingredients:

3 large oranges, wedged and deseeded

2 medium-sized carrots, sliced

1 large mango, peeled and chopped

1 tsp of ginger, ground

2 tbsp of lemon juice

½ cup of water

A few mint leaves

Preparation:

Combine all ingredients in a food processor and blend until nicely smooth. Transfer the mixture to a serving glasses and garnish with fresh mint.

Serve immediately.

Nutrition information per serving: Kcal: 131, Protein: 2.4g, Carbs: 32.2g, Fats: 0.6g

10. Black Seafood Pasta

Ingredients:

1 lb of fresh seafood mix

3 tbsp of olive oil

4 garlic cloves, crushed

1 tbsp of fresh parsley, finely chopped

1 tsp of fresh rosemary, finely chopped

½ cup of white wine

1 tsp of salt

1 lb squid ink pasta

Preparation:

Use a package instructions to prepare pasta. Squid ink pasta usually doesn't take more than five minutes in a pot of boiling water, so be careful not to overcook it. Set aside.

Preheat the oil in a deep pot over a medium-high temperature. Add garlic and briefly stir-fry for about 2-3 minutes, or until translucent. Now, add seafood mix, fresh parsley, chopped rosemary, and salt. Stir in the wine and

½ cup of water. Add more water to adjust the thickness if needed.Cover with a lid and reduce the heat to low. Cook for about 1 hour.

Stir in the previously cooked pasta and cook for 5 more minutes. Sprinkle with Parmesan before serving, but this is optional.

Nutrition information per serving: Kcal: 273, Protein: 26.1g, Carbs: 3.8g, Fats: 14.6g

11. Barbunya Pilaki

Ingredients:

2 cups of cranberry beans

2 medium-sized onions, peeled and finely chopped

3 large carrots, cleaned and chopped

3 large tomatoes, diced

3 tbsp of olive oil

A handful of fresh parsley

2 cups of water

Preparation:

Soak the beans overnight. Rinse and set aside.

Preheat the oil in a large skillet over a medium-high temperature. Add beans, carrots, tomatoes, and parsley. Pour the water and cook cover with a lid. Reduce the heat to low and cook for 2 hours. Add more water during cooking time if it is too thick. Remove from the heat and serve

Nutrition information per serving: Kcal: 329, Protein: 16.5g, Carbs: 50.9g, Fats: 8.2g

12. Apple Pie

Ingredients:

2 lbs of Zestar apples, cored, peeled and chopped

2 tbsp of honey, raw

¼ cup of breadcrumbs

2 tsp of cinnamon, ground

3 tbsp of lemon juice, freshly squeezed

1 tsp of vanilla sugar

¼ cup of oil

1 large egg, beaten

¼ cup of all-purpose flour

2 tbsp of flaxseeds

Pie dough

Preparation:

Preheat the oven to 375°F.

Combine apples and lemon juice in a large bowl. Set aside for 10 minutes.

Now add breadcrumbs, vanilla sugar,honey, and cinnamon. You can also add one teaspoon of ground nutmeg in the mixture, but this is optional. Mix well the ingredients and set aside.

On a lightly floured surface roll out the pie dough making 2 circle-shaped crusts. Take a round baking dish and grease it with the oil. Place the crust on the bottom, spoon the apple mixture, and cover with the remaining crust. Seal by crimping edges and brush with beaten egg. Sprinkle with flaxseeds and put it in the oven. Bake for 45 minutes, or until golden crisp.

Nutrition information per serving: Kcal: 214, Protein: 2.8g, Carbs: 27.4g, Fats: 11.6g

13. Green Meat Rolls

Ingredients:

1.5 lb of collard greens, steamed

1 lb lean ground beef

2 small onions, finely chopped

½ cup of white rice, long grain

2 tbsp of olive oil

1 tsp of salt

½ tsp of black pepper, ground

1 tsp of mint leaves, finely chopped

2 cups of lukewarm water

Preparation:

Boil a large pot of water and add the greens. Briefly, cook for 2-3 minutes. Drain and gently squeeze the greens and set aside.

In a large bowl, combine the ground beef with finely chopped onions, rice, salt, pepper, and mint leaves.

Preheat the oil in a large skillet over a medium-low temperature. Place leaves on your work surface, vein side up. Use one tablespoon of the meat mixture and place it in the bottom center of each leaf. Fold the sides over and roll up tightly. Tuck in the sides and gently transfer to a skillet. Repeat the process with remaining meat mixture. Add 2 cups of water and cover with a lid.

Reduce the heat to low and cook for 3 hours. Serve warm.

Nutrition information per serving: Kcal: 156, Protein: 5.2g, Carbs: 21.4g, Fats: 7.8g

14. Mackerel with Potatoes and Greens

Ingredients:

4 medium-sized mackerels, cleaned

1 lb of fresh spinach, chopped

5 large potatoes, peeled and sliced

3 tbsp of olive oil

3 garlic cloves, crushed

1 tsp of dried rosemary, finely chopped

2 springs of fresh mint leaves, chopped

1 lemon, juiced

1 tsp of sea salt

Preparation:

Combine lemon juice, rosemary, mint, salt, and pepper in a mixing bowl. Stir well and set aside.

Place the potatoes in a pot of boiling water. Cook until fork-tender and remove from the heat. Drain well and set side.

Preheat the oil in a large nonstick saucepan over a medium-high temperature. Add garlic and stir-fry until translucent. Now, add fish and grill for 5 minutes on each side, or until set. Remove the fish from the saucepan and reserve the pan. Add spinach and cook for about 2-3 minutes, or until soften. Remove from the heat.

Combine potatoes, spinach, and the fish on a serving plate. Drizzle all with marinade and serve.

Nutrition information per serving: Kcal: 244, Protein: 14.3g, Carbs: 19.2g, Fats: 12.3g

15. Chopped Veal Kebab with Butter

Ingredients:

2 lbs boneless veal shoulder, cut into bite-sized pieces

3 large tomatoes, roughly chopped

2 tbsp of all-purpose flour

3 tbsp of butter

1 tbsp of cayenne pepper

1 tsp of salt

1 tbsp of parsley, finely chopped

1 cup of Greek yogurt

1 pide bread

Preparation:

Melt 2 tablespoons of butter in a large skillet over a medium-high temperature. Add meat and sprinkle with some salt to taste. Cook for 10 minutes, or until slightly browned. Now, add water enough to cover the meat and bring it to a boil. Stir in the tomatoes and reduce the heat to low.

Meanwhile, melt the remaining butter in a saucepan over a medium-high temperature. Stir in flour, cayenne pepper, salt, and pepper. Fry for about 2-3 minutes, stirring constantly. Remove from the heat.

Chop the pide bread and place it on a serving plate. Top with meat and tomato mixture. Drizzle with previously made sauce and add yogurt on side. Sprinkle all with fresh parsley and serve.

Nutrition information per serving: Kcal: 437, Protein: 49.7g, Carbs: 8.9g, Fats: 21.8g

16. Tangerine Kale Smoothie

Ingredients:

3 cups of tangerines, wedged

2 cups of fresh kale, chopped

1 large banana, chopped

1 tsp of ginger, ground

½ cup of Greek yogurt

Preparation:

Combine all ingredients in a food processor and blend for 3 minutes, until smooth and creamy. Transfer the mixture to a serving glasses and serve immediately.

Nutrition information per serving: Kcal: 106, Protein: 3.7g, Carbs: 24.2g, Fats: 0.5g

17. Sea Fennel Pizza

Ingredients:

1 standard pizza dough

½ cup of tomato paste

¼ cup of water

1 tsp of dried oregano, ground

7 oz of button mushrooms, sliced

½ cup of Gouda cheese, grated

¼ cup of sea fennel

¼ cup of arugula, finely chopped

2 tbsp of extra virgin olive oil

¼ tsp of black pepper, ground

¼ tsp of chili pepper, ground

¼ tsp of salt

Preparation:

Preheat the oven to 450°F.

Combine tomato paste, water, chili, and oregano in a small bowl. Flour the working space and place the pizza dough on it. Spread the mixture evenly over a dough. Now, spread mushrooms and cheese and sprinkle with some parsley. You can add some more vegetables by your choice.

Take a large baking sheet and place some baking paper on it. Grease with oil and place the pizza. Place it in the oven and bake for about 15-20 minutes, or until brown and crispy. Remove from the oven and top with sea fennel and arugula.

Cut into slices and serve warm.

Nutrition information per serving: Kcal: 423, Protein: 12g, Carbs: 30.6g, Fats: 29.4g

18. Eggplant Stew

Ingredients:

4 medium-sized eggplants, halved

3 large tomatoes, finely chopped

2 red bell peppers, seeded and finely chopped

¼ cup of tomato paste

2 tbsp of fresh parsley, finely chopped

3 oz of toasted almonds, finely chopped

2 tbsp of salted capers, rinsed and drained

¼ cup of extra virgin olive oil

1 tsp of sea salt

2 tsp of granulated sugar

Preparation:

Grease the bottom of a deep pot with 2 tablespoons of extra virgin olive oil. Make the first layer with halved eggplants and tuck in the ends gently to fit in.

Now make the second layer with finely chopped tomatoes and red bell peppers. Spred the tomato paste evenly over the vegetables, sprinkle with finely chopped almonds and salted capers. Add the remaining olive oil, salt and pepper.

Pour about 1 ½ cups of water and cover the lid. Cook for about 2 hours on a low temperature.

Nutrition information per serving: Kcal: 259, Protein: 7.5g, Carbs: 30g, Fats: 15.1g

19. Cherry Pie

Ingredients:

2 cups all-purpose flour

½ tsp of salt

1 tsp of honey, raw

1 cup butter, softened

1 cup of cold water

1 lb of cherries, pitted

½ cup of cherry jam

¼ cup of cornstarch

1 tbsp of vanilla extract

1 large egg, beaten

Preparation:

Preheat the oven to 400°F.

Combine flour, salt, and honey. Mix well and add softened butter and about 1 cup of cold water. Mix well with an electric mixer or in a food processor, until dough is crumbly. Divide in half and press each portion into ½ inch thick discs. Wrap in plastic and refrigerate for about 30 minutes.

Meanwhile, combine pitted cherries with cherry jam, cornstarch, and vanilla extract. Beat well with an electric mixer on low to keep cherries whole.

Roll each disk of dough to fit a 9-inch pie plate. Cut one disc into 8-9 strips (about 1 inch each). Gently fit the dough into a pie plate and pour in the cherry mixture. Flatten the surface with a spatula and use the strips cover the pie.

Lightly brush with beaten egg and bake for about an 70-80 minutes.

Nutritional information per serving: Kcal: 641, Protein: 9.6g, Carbs: 77.2g, Fats: 32.2g

20. Strawberry Oatmeal Bars

Ingredients:

2 cups of cream cheese

½ cup of coconut oil

1 tsp strawberry extract

2 cups frozen strawberries

½ cup of oats

Preparation:

Combine cream cheese, coconut oil, strawberry extract, oats, and frozen strawberries in a large bowl. Beat well with an electric mixer until all well incorporated. Spread the mixture on a serving platter or a baking sheet. Refrigerate for 45 minutes and then cut into bars.

Keep in the refrigerator up to 10 days.

Nutrition information per serving: Kcal: 282, Protein: 6.6g, Carbs: 3.9g, Fats: 27.4g

21. Marinara Turkey

Ingredients:

1 lb of turkey breasts, cut into bite-sized pieces

1 cup of cherry tomatoes, halved

½ cup of basil, chopped

2 garlic cloves, minced

¼ cup of shallots, chopped

4 tbsp of tomato sauce

5 tbsp of olive oil

½ tsp of salt

¼ tsp of black pepper, ground

Preparation:

Combine cherry tomatoes, basil, shallots, tomato sauce, salt, pepper, and 4 tablespoons of oil in a food processor. Blend until smooth and creamy and set aside.

Preheat the remaining oil in a large nonstick frying pan over a medium-high temperature. Add garlic and stir-fry for 2 minutes. Now, add meat chops and fry for 5-7 minutes, or until nicely brown. Transfer the meat to a serving plate and drizzle with marinara sauce and serve.

Nutrition information per serving: Kcal: 290, Protein: 20.4g, Carbs: 9.7g, Fats: 19.5g

22. Green Papaya Smoothie

Ingredients:

2 cups of papaya, peeled and chopped

2 cups of spinach, chopped

1 large banana, chopped

1 cup of Greek yogurt

¼ cup of raisins, chopped

2 tbsp of flaxseeds

Preparation:

Combine all ingredients in a food processor. Blend until smooth and creamy. Transfer to a serving glasses and serve immediately.

Nutrition information per serving: Kcal: 185, Protein: 7.8g, Carbs: 34.5g, Fats: 3.0g

23. Beef Steaks in Green Puree

Ingredients:

1 lbs of beef steaks

1 cup of broccoli, chopped

1 cup of cauliflower, chopped

5 tbsp of olive oil

4 tsp of fresh parsley, finely chopped

2 cups of beef broth

1 tsp of sea salt

¼ tsp of black pepper, ground

Preparation:

Preheat the 2 tablespoons of oil in a large frying pan over a medium-high temperature. Add steaks and fry for about 5 minutes, or until browned. Remove from the heat and set aside.

Heat up the bone broth in a medium pot, but do not boil. Add cauliflower and broccoli. Add water to cover all ingredients if needed. Cook for 5 minutes on a low temperature. Transfer to a food processor, and add parsley, remaining oil, and salt. Blend until smooth and transfer to a bowl.

Serve with beef steaks as a side dish or pour over the meat.

Nutrition information per serving: Kcal: 316, Protein: 30.4g, Carbs: 2.8g, Fats: 20.3g

24. Chocolate Gingerbread Cookies

Ingredients:

1 ½ cup all-purpose flour

½ cup of honey, raw

1 tsp baking soda

½ tsp bicarbonate of soda

1 tsp of cinnamon, ground

1 tbsp of ginger, ground

1 tsp of nutmeg, ground

1 cup of butter

¼ cup molasses

1 large egg

1 cup of chocolate chips

Preparation:

Preheat the oven to 300°F.

Line two baking sheets with parchment.

Combine all dry ingredients in a large bowl. Set aside.

Chop chocolate into bite-sized chunks and set aside.

In a medium-sized bowl, combine butter with molasses, one large egg, and chocolate chips. Beat well for 3-4 minutes. Combine with flour mixture and continue to beat until well incorporated. Place dough on a clean and lightly floured surface. Flatten to 0.5 inches thick and wrap in plastic. Refrigerate for 30 minutes.

Using different shape cutters, cut out shapes and place on a baking sheet. Bake for 10-15 minutes.

Transfer to a wire rack to cool completely. Serve.

Nutrition information per serving: Kcal: 327, Protein: 6.3g, Carbs: 31.5g, Fats: 19.8g

25. Chicken with Potatoes and Leeks

Ingredients:

1 lbs of chicken breasts, cut into bite-sized pieces

2 cups of leeks, chopped

3 small potatoes, peeled and chopped

1 cup of Brussel sprouts, halved

1 cup of vegetable broth

1 cup of tomato sauce

2 tbsp of vegetable oil

2 garlic cloves, minced

½ tsp of chili pepper, ground

½ tsp of salt

Preparation:

Preheat the 1 tablespoon of oil in a large nonstick skillet over a medium-high temperature. Add meat and cook for 10 minutes, until nicely browned. Set aside.

Preheat the remaining oil in the same skillet over a medium-high temperature. Add leeks, Brussel sprouts, garlic, chili, and salt to the pan. Cook for 5 minutes, or until vegetables are fork-tender. Now, pour vegetable broth, tomato sauce, and potatoes and give it a good stir. Cook for about 25-30 minutes, or until vegetables are set. Remove from the heat and serve with meat.

Nutrition information per serving: Kcal: 244, Protein: 22.0g, Carbs: 18.5g, Fats: 9.1g

26. Lemon Smoothie

Ingredients:

½ cup of lemon juice, freshly squeezed

2 tbsp of lime juice

2 tbsp of fresh mint, chopped

1 cup of Greek yogurt

2 tbsp of honey, raw

¼ tsp of cinnamon

Preparation:

Combine all ingredients in a food processor and blend until smooth. Add a few ice cubes and re-blend for 15 seconds. Transfer the mixture to a serving glasses and garnish with some fresh mint or some extra seeds and nuts.

Nutrition information per serving: Kcal: 152, Protein: 9.8g, Carbs: 23.0g, Fats: 2.4g

27. Spicy Chicken with Broccoli

Ingredients:

1 lb of chicken breasts, skinless and boneless

2 cups of broccoli, chopped

2 tsp of chili pepper, ground

1 tsp of ginger, ground

4 garlic cloves, minced

1 tbsp of fresh parsley, finely chopped

2 tbsp of lime juice

6 tbsp of olive oil

1 tsp of sea salt

Preparation:

Preheat 2 tablespoons of oil in a large frying skillet over a medium-high temperature. Add garlic,chicken breasts, and sprinkle with parsley. Cook for 4 minutes on each side, or until nicely browned. Remove from the heat and set aside.

Combine the remaining oil, lime juice, ginger, chili, and salt in a mixing bowl. Stir well to mix and set aside.

Heat the steamer and place chopped broccoli in it. Steam for about 5-6 minutes, or until slightly soften. Transfer the broccoli to serving plate.

Serve with meat and drizzle with dressing.

Nutrition information per serving: Kcal: 419, Protein: 34.4g, Carbs: 4.7g, Fats: 29.6g

28. Protein Balls

Ingredients:

1 cup of dried figs

½ cup dried cranberries

½ cup almonds, finely chopped

¼ cup butter, chopped

2 tbsp coconut oil

1 tsp vanilla sugar

1 tbsp chia seeds

½ tsp of cinnamon, ground

1 tbsp of ginger, ground

2 tbsp of flaxseed

1 tbsp of molasses

Preparation:

Combine all ingredients in a medium-sized bowl. Mix well with a spoon or with an electric mixer. Roll into bite-sized balls and coat in shredded coconut.

Keep in the refrigerator up to 7 days.

Nutrition information per serving: Kcal: 173, Protein: 4.2g, Carbs: 17.4g, Fats: 10.5g

29. Braised Kale

Ingredients:

10 oz of kale, chopped

2 small onions, finely chopped

2 garlic cloves, crushed

1 tsp of red chili pepper, ground

4 tbsp of butter

2 cups of vegetable broth

1 tsp of salt

1 tbsp of lemon juice

Preparation:

Melt the butter in a large saucepan over a medium-high temperature. Add onions, garlic and red pepper. Stir-fry for 5 minutes or until translucent.

Now, pour the broth and stir in the kale. Sprinkle with salt and cover with a lid. Reduce the heat to low and cook for 40 minutes.

Remove from the heat and sprinkle with lemon juice before serving.

Nutrition information per serving: Kcal: 174, Protein: 5.2g, Carbs: 11.9g, Fats: 12.3g

30. Chili Tuna Wraps

Ingredients:

4 cans of Albacore tuna, drained

2 medium-sized cucumbers, finely chopped

4 tbsp of shallots, chopped

½ cup of frozen corn, thawed

4 tbsp of mayonnaise

1 tbsp of lemon juice

½ tsp of salt

¼ tsp of black pepper, ground

½ small chili pepper, minced

6 large lettuce leaves

Preparation:

Combine all ingredients except lettuce leaves in a large bowl. Toss well to combine and set aside for 20 minutes to allow flavors to meld.

Spread the lettuce leaves on a clean surface and spoon the mixture. Wrap and secure with a toothpick. Serve immediately.

Nutrition information per serving: Kcal: 142, Protein: 16.7g, Carbs: 10.6g, Fats: 4.5g

31. Chocolate Protein Muffins

Ingredients:

1 ½ cup all-purpose flour

½ cup of cocoa powder, raw

1 tsp of baking powder

1 tsp vanilla sugar

½ cup of honey, raw

2 large eggs

1 cup of skim milk

3 tbsp vegetable oil

Preparation:

Preheat oven to 325°F.

Line one 6-cup muffin tins with paper liners.

Combine all dry ingredients in a large bowl. In another bowl, gently whisk together eggs, honey, milk, ½ cup of lukewarm water, and oil. Using an electric mixer, beat until well incorporated. Now add the flour mixture and continue beating until smooth mixture.

Using a spoon or ice cream scoop, divide the mixture evenly among the tins. Bake for 20-30 or until the toothpick inserted into the middle comes out clean. Let it cool for another 30 minutes.

Optionally, sprinkle muffins with shredded coconut and serve.

Nutrition information per serving: Kcal: 143, Protein: 5.9g, Carbs: 15.9g, Fats: 7.3g

32. Juicy Venison Steaks

Ingredients:

4 medium-sized venison steaks, boneless

1 cup of butter

2 tbsp of lemon juice

2 garlic cloves, minced

1 large onion, chopped

2 tbsp of balsamic vinegar

2 large bell peppers, chopped

2 tsp of salt

½ tsp of black pepper, ground

Preparation:

Place the meat in a large bowl. Add salt and coat well. Set aside for 20 minutes.

Melt the butter in a large nonstick frying pan over a medium-high temperature. Add onions and garlic and stir-fry for 2 minutes. Now, add meat and fry for 3-4 minutes on each side, or until browned. Remove the meat to a serving plate, but reserve the pan.

Add bell peppers, vinegar, lemon juice, salt, and pepper to the frying pan. Stir and cook until simmer. Remove from the heat and drizzle the meat with this mixture. Serve immediately.

Nutrition information per serving: Kcal: 596, Protein: 31.6g, Carbs: 8.9g, Fats: 48.6g

33. Red Pepper Pesto

Ingredients:

2 large red bell peppers, seeded and halved

1 cup of Ricotta cheese

¼ cup of almonds, roughly chopped

3 tbsp of tomato paste

1 garlic clove, minced

1 tsp of dried oregano, ground

4 tbsp of olive oil

1 tsp of salt

½ tsp of chili pepper, ground

Preparation:

Preheat the oven to 375°F.

Grease a large baking sheet with 2 tablespoons of oil. Spread the peppers and put it in the oven. Bake for about 20 minutes, or until charcoal crisp. Remove from the oven and set aside to cool for a while.

Peel off the skin and place in a food processor. Add all other ingredients and blend until nicely smooth. Store the pesto in a jar and refrigerate.

Serve with pasta or rice.

Nutrition information per serving: Kcal: 181, Protein: 6.4g, Carbs: 7.8g, Fats: 14.8g

34. Coconut Grapefruit Smoothie

Ingredients:

1 medium-sized grapefruit, peeled and chopped

1 large banana, chopped

2 cups of Romaine lettuce

1 tsp of ginger, ground

1 cup of coconut milk

1 tbsp of honey, raw

1 tbsp of coconut, shredded

Preparation:

Combine all ingredients except shredded coconut in a food processor. Blend until smooth and transfer to a serving glasses. Sprinkle with shredded coconut and serve immediately.

Nutrition information per serving: Kcal: 214, Protein: 2.4g, Carbs: 21.9g, Fats: 15.0g

35. Green Sunflower Salad

Ingredients:

2 cups of arugula, chopped

2 cups of Iceberg lettuce, chopped

1 cup of red cabbage, shredded

1 small onion, sliced

1 tbsp of sunflower seeds

3 tbsp of extra-virgin olive oil

1 tbsp of lemon juice

1 tbsp of orange juice

1 tsp of lemon zest

1 tbsp of honey, raw

½ tsp of salt

¼ tsp of black pepper, ground

Preparation:

Mix together oil, lemon juice, orange juice, honey, salt, and pepper in a mixing bowl. Set aside for 10 minutes to allow flavors to meld.

Wash and cut all vegetables and combine in a large salad bowl. Mix with a spoon and then add sunflower seeds. Drizzle with dressing and stir well to combine. Serve immediately.

Nutrition information per serving: Kcal: 262, Protein: 2.1g, Carbs: 18.0g, Fats: 22.2g

36. Coconut Porridge

Ingredients:

1 cup of coconut, shredded

2 cups of oatmeal

½ cup of almonds, roughly chopped

½ cup of coconut milk

2 tbsp of coconut oil

1 tsp of cinnamon, ground

1 cup of water

Preparation:

Preheat the oven to 325°F.

Combine coconut oil and cinnamon in a fire-proof bowl. Melt in a microwave oven. Add oatmeals and soak for 10 minutes. Stir few times during soaking process.

Take a small baking dish or a casserolle dish and line some baking paper. Spread the mixture evenly and place it in the oven. Bake for about 2-3 minutes and remove from the oven. Return the mixture to the bowl and pour the coconut milk and water. Stir all well to combine and serve.

Nutrition information per serving: Kcal: 565, Protein: 12.4g, Carbs: 47.2g, Fats: 39.0g

37. Chicken Tacos

Ingredients:

1 lbs of chicken thighs, skinless and chopped

2 cups of spring onions, chopped

2 medium-sized bell peppers, chopped

1 cup of sour cream

1 cup of chicken broth

2 tbsp of olive oil

1 tsp of chili pepper, ground

1 tbsp of sweet paprika, ground

½ tsp of salt

¼ tsp of black pepper, ground

A handful of spinach leaves, whole

Preparation:

Preheat 1 tablespoon of oil in a large saucepan over a medium-high temperature. Add the meat and sprinkle with some salt. Fry for 10 minutes, or until brown and crisp. Remove from the heat and set aside. Reserve the pan.

Add the remaining oil to the saucepan. Add spring onions and bell peppers. Pout the broth and sprinkle with sweet paprika, chili, and pepper. Stir all well and cook until simmer.

Stir in the meat and sour cream and reduce the heat to low. Cook for about 5 minutes more and remove from the heat.

Spread a small bunch of spinach leaves over a serving plate and spoon the meat mixture. Serve.

Nutrition information per serving: Kcal: 299, Protein: 25.1g, Carbs: 8.0g, Fats: 18.8g

38. Orange Carrot Soup

Ingredients:

5 large oranges, diced

1 lb of carrots, grated

1 small onion, diced

½ cup of vegetable broth

½ cup of Greek yogurt

2 small potatoes, peeled and chopped

1 tbsp of coriander, ground

1 tsp of ginger, ground

2 tbsp of vegetable oil

½ tsp of salt

½ tsp of black pepper, ground

Preparation:

Preheat the oil in a large skillet over a medium-high temperature. Add the onion and stir-fry for 2-3 minutes or until translucent.

Add vegetable broth, carrots, ginger, and coriander. Bring it to a boil and remove from the heat. Transfer the mixture to a food processor and sprinkle with salt and pepper. Blend until smooth and return to the skillet. Stir in the oranges and yogurt and heat it up.

Remove from the heat and serve.

Nutrition information per serving: Kcal: 151, Protein: 3.7g, Carbs: 27.3g, Fats: 3.9g

39. Hot Pistachio Cereals

Ingredients:

1 cup of oatmeal

1 cup of water, boiled

3 tbsp of pistachios, unsalted

1 tsp of pistachios, grated

1 cup of Greek yogurt

2 tbsp of honey, liquid

Preparation:

Combine water and oatmeal in a medium pot over a medium-high temperature. Bring it to a boil and remove from the heat. Set aside to cool completely. Transfer to a serving dishes.

Now, rougly chop pistachios and add it to the oatmeal. Stir well and top with yogurt. Sprinkle with grated pistachios for some extra taste.

Nutrition information per serving: Kcal: 214, Protein: 10.5g, Carbs: 33.5g, Fats: 4.9g

40. Salmon Balsamico

Ingredients:

2 lbs of salmon fillets, skinless and boneless

1 cup of balsamic vinegar

½ cup of shallots, chopped

2 garlic cloves, minced

1 small onion, diced

1 tbsp of honey, raw

2 tbsp of olive oil

2 tbsp of lemon juice

2 tbsp of parsley, finely chopped

½ tsp of salt

½ tsp of black pepper, freshly ground

Preparation:

Preheat 1 tablespoon of oil in a large nonstick skillet over a medium-high temperature. Add the onions and garlic and stir-fry for 3 minutes, or until translucent. Stir in the shallots, vinegar, lemon juice, parsley, and honey. Reduce the heat to low and cook for about 3-4 minutes. Remove from the heat and set aside.

Meanwhile, preheat the remaining oil in a nonstick frying pan over a medium-high temperature. Add the fillets and fry for 4-5 minutes on each side. Remove from the heat and transfer to a serving plate and drizzle with vinegar sauce.

Nutrition information per serving: Kcal: 277, Protein: 30.0g, Carbs: 7.2g, Fats: 14.1g

41. Basmati Rice with Curry

Ingredients:

2 cups od basmati rice

1 cup of spring onions, chopped

2 garlic cloves, minced

1 small red onion, chopped

1 tbsp of curry powder

1 small chili pepper, finely chopped

½ cup of parsley, finely chopped

1 cup of raisins

¼ cup of red wine vinegar

2 tbsp of lemon juice

1 tsp of salt

¼ tsp of black pepper, ground

Preparation:

Place the rice in a deep pot and add about 4 cups of water. Cover with a lid and bring it to a boil. Reduce the temperature to low and continue to cook for 45 minutes.

Meanwhile, combine all other ingredients in a large mixing bowl. Stir well and set aside while rice is cooking.

Remove the rice from the heat set aside to cool for a while. Stir in the rice into the bowl and sprinkle with more salt or pepper, if needed.

Serve immediately.

Nutrition information per serving: Kcal: 476, Protein: 8.9g, Carbs: 108.4g, Fats: 1.2g

42. Dates Muesli

Ingredients:

1 cup of rolled oats

1 cup of dates, pitted and chopped

1 large banana, sliced

1 cup of coconut milk

¼ tsp of cinnamon, ground

1 tbsp of honey, raw

1 tbsp of almonds, roughly chopped

Preparation:

Combine rolled oats, dates, banana, and honey in a medium bowl. Stir in coconut milk and sprinkle with cinnamon for some extra taste. Set aside for 20 minutes before serving.

Nutrition information per serving: Kcal: 528, Protein: 7.8g, Carbs: 84.1g, Fats: 22.2g

43. Eggplant Puree & Marinated Tomato Wraps

Ingredients:

1 large eggplant, peeled and chopped

2 tbsp of tahini

½ tsp of cumin, ground

3 garlic cloves, minced

2 tbsp of lemon juice, freshly squeezed

½ tsp of salt

¼ tsp of Cayenne pepper, ground

¼ tsp of black pepper, ground

7 Iceberg lettuce leaves

For the tomatoes:

3 medium-sized tomatoes, diced

2 garlic cloves, minced

3 tbsp of balsamic vinegar

1 tbsp of olive oil

¼ tsp of salt

Preparation:

Preheat the oven to 400°F.

Take a large baking sheet and line some parchment paper. Spread the eggplant chops and sprinkle with some salt to taste. Bake for about 45 minutes, or until tender. Remove from the heat and let it cool.

Transfer the eggplant to the food processor. Add all other ingredients gradually and blend until smooth. Set aside.

Combine vinegar, oil, garlic, salt and pepper in a medium bowl. Add tomatoes and toss to coat well.

Place one large lettuce leaf over a serving plate. Spoon 1 tablespoon of eggplant puree, then 1 tablespoon of marinated tomatoes. Wrap and secure with a toothpick. Serve immediately.

Nutrition information per serving: Kcal: 185, Protein: 2.2g, Carbs: 9.2g, Fats: 4.7g

44. Spicy Tomato Smoothie

Ingredients:

1 large tomato, diced

1 large bell pepper, seeded and chopped

½ cup of zucchini, chopped

1 cup of celery, finely chopped

1 tbsp of flaxseeds

½ tsp of chili pepper, ground

¼ tsp of Cayenne pepper, ground

Preparation:

Combine all ingredients in a food processor and blend until nicely smooth. Transfer to a serving glasses and set aside for 15 minutes before serving.

Nutrition information per serving: Kcal: 68, Protein: 2.8g, Carbs: 11.8g, Fats: 1.6g

45. Fava Beans

Ingredients:

1 lb of fava beans, soaked overnight

2 small onions, diced

2 garlic cloves, minced

1 tsp of cumin, ground

3 tbsp of lemon juice, freshly squeezed

1 tbsp of olive oil

¼ tsp of salt

¼ tsp of chili pepper, ground

¼ tsp of black pepper, ground

Preparation:

Soak the beans for at least 10 hours, or overnight.

Drain and rinse the beans with cold water. Place them in a large pot and add water enough to cover it. Bring it to a boil over a medium-high temperature. Now, reduce the heat to low and cook for 2 hours, or until soften. Drain half of the liquid and set aside.

Meanwhile, preheat the oil in a large saucepan over a medium-high temperature. Stir-fry for 5 minutes, or until translucent. Stir in the cumin, and lemon juice and cook for another 3-4 minutes. Pour this mixture to the pot with beans. Add chili pepper, salt, and peppe to taste. Stir and cook for 2 more minutes. Remove from the heat and add more spices if you like.

Serve as a side with meat, or as a main dish with some lemon wedges.

Nutrition information per serving: Kcal: 544, Protein: 40.4g, Carbs: 93.9g, Fats: 2.7g

46. Turkey Artichoke Rigatoni Pasta

Ingredients:

1 lb of turkey fillets, cut into bite-sized pieces

2 cups of artichokes, chopped

1 lb of rigatoni pasta, pre-cooked

1 cup of green olives, pitted and halved

2 medium-sized tomatoes, diced

2 tbsp of tomato paste

3 garlic cloves, finely chopped

¼ cup of red wine vinegar

1 tsp of dried oregano, ground

¼ cup of fresh parsley, finely chopped

½ tsp of salt

¼ tsp of black pepper, ground

1 tbsp of vegetable oil

Preparation:

Cook the pasta according to the package instructions. Drain well and set aside.

Preheat the oil in a large skillet over a medium-high temperature. Add garlic and stir-fry for 1 minute, the add meat chops. Fry for about 8-10 minutes, or until nicely browned. Remove the meat and garlic from the skillet.

Add tomatoes, tomato paste, vinegar, and oregano to the same pan. You can add 2-3 tablespoons of water to prevent sticking. Cook for another 10 minutes, then reduce the temperature to low. Add artichokes, rigatoni, and olives. Cook for 5 minutes and sprinkle with some salt and pepper to taste. Remove from the heat and garnish with parsley before serving.

Nutrition information per serving: Kcal: 310, Protein: 24.6g, Carbs: 37.0g, Fats: 6.9g

47. Fig Spread Dessert

Ingredients:

1 cup of vegetable oil

1 cup of milk

1 cup of lukewarm water

½ cup of fig spread

1 ½ cup of all-purpose flour

½ cup of wheat groats

½ cup of corn flour

2 tsp of baking powder

Topping:

2 cups of brown sugar

2 cups of water

½ cup of fig spread

Preparation:

First, you will have to prepare the topping because it has to chill well before using it. Place sugar, fig spread, and water in a heavy bottomed pot. Bring it to a boil over medium-high heat and cook for 5 minutes, stirring constantly. Remove from the heat and cool well.

In another pot, combine oil with lukewarm water, milk, and the fig spread. Bring it to a boil and then add flour, wheat groats, corn flour, and baking powder. Give it a good stir and mix well continue to cook for 3-4 more minutes. Chill well and form the dough.

Using your hands, shape 2 inches thick balls. This mixture should give you about 16 balls, depending on the size you want. In a large baking dish, place some parchment paper and grease with some cooking spray or oil. Gently flatten the surface and transfer to a baking dish.

Bake for about 40-45 minutes and remove from the oven and let it cool for a while. Pour the cold topping over them. Refrigerate for about an hour and serve.

Nutrition information per serving: Kcal: 253, Protein: 2.2g, Carbs: 30.6g, Fats: 14.2g

48. Chicken with Quinoa

Ingredients:

2 cups of chicken breasts, chopped

1 cup of artichokes, chopped

1 cup of quinoa

1 cup of water

1 tsp of vegetable oil

1 garlic clove, minced

1 large tomato, diced

1 cup of shallots, finely chopped

¼ cup of Feta cheese, crumbled

2 tbsp of lemon juice

1 tsp of dried oregano, ground

½ tsp of salt

¼ tsp of black pepper, ground

Preparation:

Place quinoa and water in a deep pot. Bring it to a boil over a medium-high temperature. Reduce the heat to low, and cook for 10-15 minutes more. Remove from the heat and fluff with a fork. Set aside.

Preheat the oil in a large nonstick saucepan over a medium-low temperature. Add the shallots and chicken and cook for about 5-7 minutes, or until chicken is light brown.

Now, add all other ingredients and give it a good stir. Cook for another 5 minutes or until all well incorporated.

Serve warm.

Nutrition information per serving: Kcal: 275, Protein: 21.3g, Carbs: 27.7g, Fats: 9.0g

49. Beef Cutlets with Kale

Ingredients:

2 lbs of beef, minced

4 cups of fresh kale, chopped

4 large eggs

3 garlic cloves, minced

1 medium-sized red onion, chopped

1 tbsp of rosemary, finely chopped

1 tbsp of parsley, finely chopped

1 tsp of salt

1 tsbp of vegetable oil

¼ tsp of black pepper, ground

Preparation:

Preheat the oven to 400°F.

Place the kale in a pot of boiling water. Sprinkle with some salt and cook for 10 minutes, or until tender. Remove from the heat and drain well. Set aside.

Meanwhile, combine meat, eggs, garlic, onion, rosemary, parsley, salt, and pepper in a large bowl. Mix with hands and make a round-shaped cutlets, aproximately palm-sized.

Take a large baking dish and brush it with oil. Place the cutlets and kale into the dish. Bake for 35 minutes, or until well browned. Remove from the oven to cool for a while. Sprinkle with freshly squeezed lemon juice for some extra taste.

Nutrition information per serving: Kcal: 215, Protein: 44.4g, Carbs: 6.5g, Fats: 11.0g

50. Spicy Spring Omelet

Ingredients:

4 large eggs

½ cup of spring onions, chopped

½ cup of cream cheese

1 tbsp of butter

1 tsp of Himalayan salt

¼ tsp of black pepper, ground

¼ tsp of chili pepper, ground

Preparation

Combine eggs, cheese, onions, salt, pepper, and chili in a medium bowl. Mix well until incorporated. Set aside.

Melt the butter in a large nonstick frying pan over a medium-high temperature. Pour the omelet and cook for 3 minutes, then flip and cook another 3 minutes on the other side. Fold the omelet and serve immediately.

Nutrition information per serving: Kcal: 405, Protein: 17.5g, Carbs: 4.4g, Fats: 36.0g

51. Macadamia Crepes

Ingredients:

½ cup of macadamia nuts, chopped

4 large eggs, beaten

½ cup of skim milk

½ cup of sour cream

1 tsp of baking soda

1 tsp of cinnamon, ground

1 tbsp of coconut oil

4 tsp of cocoa powder, raw

Preparation:

Combine nuts, baking soda, cinnamon, and cocoa in a large mixing bowl. Stir well and then add milk, eggs, and sour cream. Use a hand mixer to make nice batter mixture.

Melt the coconut oil in a frying pan over a medium-low temperature. Add about 2-3 tablespoons of batter to the pan and spread evenly. Fry for about 5-7 minutes and flip the crepes. Fry 1-2 minutes on the other side and remove from the heat.

Spread the fruit jam melted chocolate and roll the crepes before serving.

Nutrition information per serving: Kcal: 399, Protein: 13.2g, Carbs: 9.2g, Fats: 36.4g

52. Creamy Roasted Asparagus

Ingredients:

2 lbs of asparagus, trimmed

2 tbsp of olive oil

1 cup of sour cream

½ cup of parmesan cheese

2 tbsp of lemon juice

1 tsp of sea salt

1 tsp of rosemary, finely chopped

¼ tsp of black pepper, ground

Preparation:

Preheat the oven to 400°F.

Mix together sour cream, 1 tablespoon of oil, lemon juice, salt, rosemary, and pepper in a medium bowl. Stir all well to combine and set aside.

Take a large baking dish and grease with the remaining oil. Spread the asparagus evenly. Place in the oven and and bake for 10 minutes, or until slighltly tender. Shake the pan occasionally to stir the asparagus. Now, pour the cream mixture and return to oven for another 3 minutes. Remove from the oven and let it cool for a while. Sprinkle with Parmesan and some extra black pepper to taste.

Nutrition information per serving: Kcal: 197, Protein: 8.9g, Carbs: 8.3g, Fats: 15.8g

53. Spicy Egg Vegetable Salad

Ingredients:

1 cup of fresh celery, chopped

1 cup of tomatoes, chopped

½ cup of cucumber, sliced

1 cup of Romaine lettuce, chopped

½ cup of spring onions, chopped

2 large eggs, hard-boiled

5 tbsp of lemon juice

1 tbsp of garlic, minced

½ tsp of vegetable seasoning mix

½ tsp of salt

¼ tsp of black pepper, ground

Preparation:

Mix together lemon juice, garlic, vegetable seasoning mix, salt, and pepper ina mixing bowl. Stir well and set aside.

Gently place the eggs in a pot of boiling water. Cook for 5 minutes and remove from the heat. Drain in cold water and peel. Chop the eggs in wedges and place in a large bowl. Add tomatoes, celer, cucumber, lettuce, and spring onions.

Drizzle with dressing and toss well to coat. Sprinkle with chili pepper and serve immediately.

Nutrition information per serving: Kcal: 85, Protein: 8.9g, Carbs: 7.6g, Fats: 3.8g

54. Asian Beef Stew

Ingredients:

1 lb of lean beef, cut into bite-sized pieces

1 cup of coconut milk

2 tbsp of butter

½ tsp of curry, ground

¼ tsp of red pepper, ground

1 tsp of sweet paprika, ground

¼ tsp of cinnamon, ground

½ tsp of black pepper, ground

1 garlic clove, minced

½ tsp of salt

Preparation:

Melt the butter in a large nonstick skillet over a medium-high temperature. Add meat and cook for 10 minutes, or until golden brown.

Now, reduce the temperature to low and add coconut milk. Sprinkle with curry, red pepper, paprika, cinnamon, garlic, black pepper, and salt. Stir all well to combine and cover with a lid. Cook for 2 hours. If the liquid evaporates, add more water. Stir occasionally.

Serve warm with steamed vegetables or rice.

Nutrition information per serving: Kcal: 406, Protein: 36.1g, Carbs: 4.9g, Fats: 27.3g

55. Lemon Oatmeal

Ingredients:

1 cup of cream cheese

1 cup of oatmeal

¼ cup of heavy cream

5 tbsp of lemon juice, freshly squeezed

2 tbsp of honey, raw

1 tsp of lemon zest, freshly grated

Preparation:

Combine cream cheese, heavy cream, and lemon juice in a medium bowl. Using hand mixer, blend all until smooth and combined.

Add oatmeal and stir with spoon until mixed. Transfer to a serving dishes. Top with honey and sprinkle with lemon zest for extra taste.

Serve immediately.

Nutrition information per serving: Kcal: 685, Protein: 14.8g, Carbs: 49.5g, Fats: 49.0g

56. Portobello Mushrooms with Arugula

Ingredients:

3 large Portobello mushrooms

4 cups of arugula, chopped

1 cup of tomatoes, sun-dried

½ tsp of dried rosemary, ground

1 tbsp of red wine vinegar

4 tbsp of olive oil

¼ tsp black pepper, ground

½ tsp of salt

Preparation:

Preheat the oven to 450°F.

Combine oil, vinegar, rosemary, and salt in mixing bowl. Stir well to combine and set aside for 5 minutes to allow flavors to mingle.

Place the mushrooms in a large bowl and pour over the marinade. Let it soak for 30 minutes. Transfer the mushrooms to a large baking dish and reserve the marinade for later.

Place it in the oven and bake for for about 10-15 minutes. Remove from the heat and place on the serving plate with arugula. Drizzle all with reserved marinade. Top with tomatoes and serve.

Nutrition information per serving: Kcal: 240, Protein: 4.1g, Carbs: 7.7g, Fats: 28.7g

ADDITIONAL TITLES FROM THIS AUTHOR

70 Effective Meal Recipes to Prevent and Solve Being Overweight: Burn Fat Fast by Using Proper Dieting and Smart Nutrition

By

Joe Correa CSN

48 Acne Solving Meal Recipes: The Fast and Natural Path to Fixing Your Acne Problems in Less Than 10 Days!

By

Joe Correa CSN

41 Alzheimer's Preventing Meal Recipes: Reduce or Eliminate Your Alzheimer's Condition in 30 Days or Less!

By

Joe Correa CSN

70 Effective Breast Cancer Meal Recipes: Prevent and Fight Breast Cancer with Smart Nutrition and Powerful Foods

By

Joe Correa CSN

www.ingramcontent.com/pod-product-compliance
Lightning Source LLC
Chambersburg PA
CBHW051030030426

42336CB00015B/2797